Mindful Eating

How to Eat Less

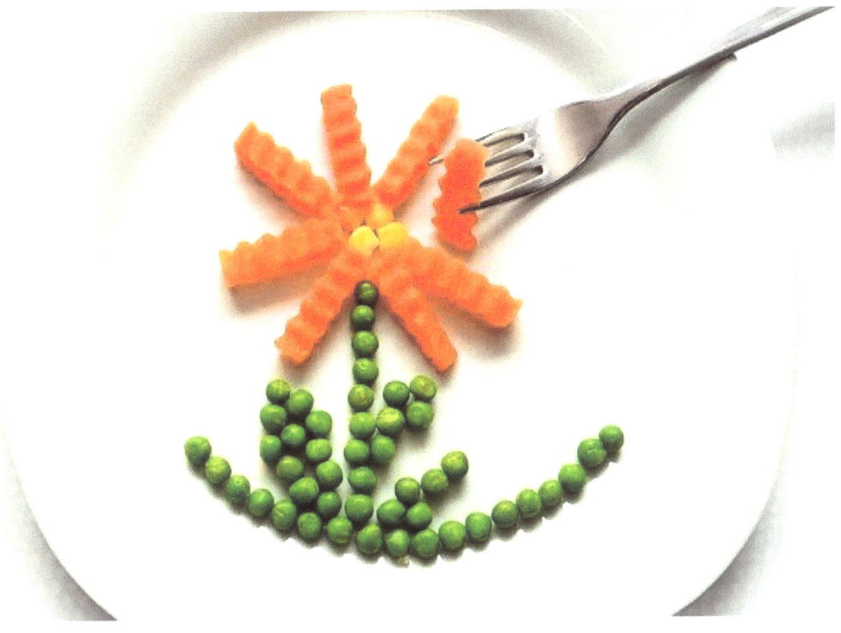

Health Learning Series

M. Usman

Mendon Cottage Books

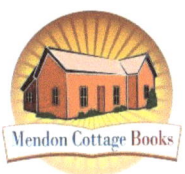

JD-Biz Publishing

Disclaimer

The information is this book is provided for informational purposes only. It is not intended to be used and medical advice or a substitute for proper medical treatment by a qualified health care provider. The information is believed to be accurate as presented based on research by the author.

The contents have not been evaluated by the U.S. Food and Drug Administration or any other Government or Health Organization and the contents in this book are not to be used to treat cure or prevent disease.

The author or publisher is not responsible for the use or safety of any diet, procedure, or treatment mentioned in this book. The author or publisher is not responsible for errors or omissions that may exist.

Warning

The Book is for informational purposes only and before taking on any diet, treatment, or medical procedure, it is recommended to consult with your primary health care provider.

Our books are available at

1. Amazon.com
2. Barnes and Noble
3. Itunes
4. Kobo
5. Smashwords
6. Google Play Books

Table of Contents

Introduction

With the revolution in cooking ingredients and networking, where we can easily share and make recipes of different states, countries, and continents just to satisfy our taste buds and have variety, there is no doubt we crave for something different every day. A new recipe, a new spice, or a new taste not only makes us crave for more, but results in mindless eating without even thinking how much harm the food will do to us and to our digestive system. The result of which has been obesity and a number of diseases.

Beyond this, the researchers and nutritionists have been following some simple tips and tricks and exercises, which not only help us enjoy all the flavors of the food, but also help us in controlling our portion size and motivating us to eat in a proper manner.

The following eBook helps us understand the concept of mindful eating, its benefits, simple tips, and exercises for eating mindfully. It also gives us an insight into the food transit time, type of over eater we are, and helps us to work towards eating less and appropriate food, as per our needs and habits.

Mindful Eating

Chapter #1: What is Mindful Eating and What are the Benefits

Mindful means "Awareness," i.e. awareness of whatever we are consuming. This awareness of food can be related to smell, taste, quality, quantity, appearance, nutritional value, and so on and so forth.

Being aware of what we intake, not only helps us control our diet, but also helps us in following a healthy lifestyle.

Benefits of mindful eating:

- **Builds a healthy lifestyle:** Structured or mindful eating helps in improving our overall relationship with food, by helping a person to eat in a balanced and conscious way, thus building a healthy lifestyle.

- **Decreases digestive problems:** Controlled eating or eating with awareness can decrease all the health hazards that are caused by unconscious eating. This unconscious eating not only disrupts our body-mind connection, but also makes our digestive system less effective; thus contributing to multiple digestive problems of gas, bloating, and bowel irregularities.

- **Weight management:** Mindful eating is "Eating with Attention and Intention." For example, when full attention is given to food, it not only helps in satisfaction and fullness by consumption of less food, but also helps in overall weight control by avoiding overeating.

- **Pleasure of eating:** When a person knows what he is eating, he not only becomes internally satisfied, but will also find more pleasure in eating.

- **Knowing your inner self:** Controlled eating helps in monitoring our senses, thus helping a person to know more about their body, soul, and mind.

- **Healing of psychological disorders:** Mindful eating, when practiced regularly, helps to avoid "emotional eating" (when a person either eats more or less because of an overflow of emotions), which may lead to problems, like obesity and depression.

- **Overall satisfaction:** Structured eating engages all parts of us—our body, heart and mind—in selecting, preparing, and eating food. It allows us to be playful about the different colors, textures, smells, tastes, and even sounds of eating and drinking. Therefore, it increases our pleasure and satisfaction of our inner cues to hunger.

Overeaters

Chapter #2: Types of Overeaters

Overeaters can be divided broadly under three categories:

1) **Feasters:** These are the people who eat too much and never feel full, because of the low production of a hormone that triggers the feeling of fullness to the brain.

2) **Cravers:** These are the people who think constantly about food. They have low resistance to curb their cravings.

3) **Emotional Eaters:** This group is for people who eat as a reaction to their feelings or during the emotional overflow periods.

So, it's important to learn which category you belong to before working on a plan of fasting, dieting, or controlled eating habits.

The following is a small quiz that will help you to get an insight into the category you belong to:

Which category of eater do you belong to?

1.   Is food always on your mind?

2.   While cooking, do you feel tempted to eat something?

3.   While passing a plate of chips or biscuits or snacks, do you usually pick one?

4.   Do you feel hungry all the time and crave to eat something constantly?

5.   Do you eat more when you are lonely?

6. Do you eat more when you are stressed?

7. Do you eat more when you are excited or anxious?

8. Do you eat more and is your eating speed high when you are angry?

9. Do you eat large potions at a time?

10. When at a party/restaurant, do your friends seem to get full earlier than you do?

11. At the end of the meal, do you still feel that you haven't had enough?

12. Whenever you start eating, do you feel you cannot stop even if you have had enough?

If the answer to questions 1-4 is a "YES," you are a "Constant Craver." If the answer to questions 5-8 is a "YES," you are an "Emotional Eater." If the answer to questions 9-12 is "YES," you are a "Feaster." If you answered "YES" to questions in different categories, you are probably a combination of more than one category.

Chapter #3: Food Preferences for Different Overeaters

Food preferences for categories:

Feasters: These people cannot stop eating in a single sitting. Since these people do not secrete enough hormones from their gut to let their brains know that they are full, a high protein and a low GI diet suits them the best.

Their food usually takes longer to digest, so it's better to have high protein foods, such as, green, leafy vegetables. They should also replace high GI foods, like white rice, white bread, pasta, and cakes with their low GI alternatives, like brown rice, whole wheat breads and pastas.

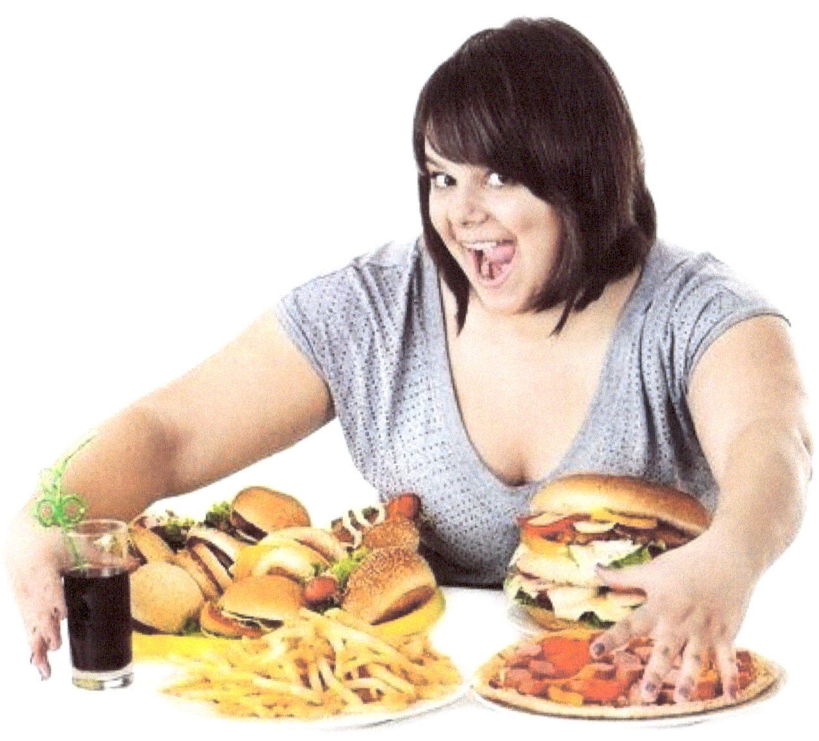

Constant cravers: These people enjoy food above anything and are at the highest risk for obesity. So, if one of your joys in life is food, what can you do to shed those extra pounds?

Intermittent fasting (two out of seven days) seems to be the only solution for them, as well as bringing on healthy alternatives on regular days.

So basically, people under this category need to change their eating habits to improve their lifestyle, and on two days when they are fasting, they need to intake no more than 800 calories.

Emotional eaters: People in this group use food to self-medicate, be it the times of high stress, anxiety, crisis, or excitement. The key to help these people is to support them in their emotional problems, which drive them to eat without even realizing how much they have eaten. Structured diets and knowing how much food should be eaten should be the base of their weight loss regime.

More than one category: There are people who love eating and are also emotional eaters. Also, there may be people who are feasters as well as emotional eaters. One may also fall under all three categories. In such cases, you need to analyze and try a couple of diets before hitting on the right kind of diet.

Over and above whatever you like to eat, you can keep those things in your diet, but just decrease the portion size and increase the portions of healthy foods, like vegetables, fruits, proteins, whole foods, etc. This will teach your brain how to eat healthier. In a way, it quenches your cravings by having foods you love in small portions and motivates you to live a healthier lifestyle.

Food Transit Time

Chapter #4: Food Transit Time

The time it takes for your food to absorb into your system, travel through your small and large intestines and then exit your body, is called the food transit time. 12-18 hours id the best rang for your food transit time. Of course, this varies for each person, but this is the normal of a healthy person.

How to measure your transit time:

One way to measure your food transit time is to eat foods that are easily visible in your stool. There are various methods in which it can be calculated, even at home.

1. Since corn is not usually completely digested, it makes it a great food to try, when testing your transit time. Corn is also a bright color which makes it visible with just a glance. You can also try sunflower seeds, if you are not a fan of corn. Make sure you write down the time you eat the corn or sunflower seeds, and also write down the time that you have a bowel movement, where the food is present.

2. Since beetroot contains a red pigment, it is also ideal to try this for timing your food transit time. Just make sure not chew it completely, so it will show up in your stool.

Short transit time (less than 10 hours): A short transit time can be caused from an intestinal infection, a food allergy, stress, hyperthyroidism, or anxiety, among other issues. A short transit time occurs when your gastrointestinal system is not functioning properly. Therefore, there is not adequate time for your body to digest and absorb nutrients.

The malabsorption of nutrients can easily cause someone suffer from malnutrition.

Long food transit time (more than 28 hours): If you eat a large amount of refined or processed foods, it can contribute to a long food transit time. A few other causes could be dehydration, lack of fiber in your diet, insufficient salt intake, hypothyroidism, and insufficient digestive enzymes.

If you are constantly going between constipation and diarrhea, you might have inflammation in the intestine. Multiple things can cause this, however the most popular are food allergies or the absence of healthy intestinal flora.

What it says about your health?

Somewhere between 12-18 hours with the maximum amount of time up to 24 hours is the best time period for your food transit time. Therefore, you should be having a bowel movement every day. But, a daily bowel movement sometimes does not necessarily tell about colon health, as even if you have a daily bowel movement, you may still have a slow transit time or could be suffering from constipation. This is the main reason you should do a bowel transit test, as you may not know if you are eliminating something that you ate two or three days before.

The longer it takes to for your food to travel through your bowels, the more time the toxins and have to wreak havoc on your body. A bowel transit time of more than 48 hours, increases the risk many diseases, including many types of cancer. You are also more susceptible to other bacterial infections, thus weakening the overall immune system. A long transit time means toxins and wastes are recirculating back to the blood stream, resulting in fatigue, headaches, acne, allergies, muscle pain, joint pains, gas, bloating, etc. A long transit time also means that a lot of fat is being absorbed from your food, leading to greater weight gain.

If you have a short transit time, it may lead to nutritional deficiencies. With a short transit time it means that your food is passing too quickly through your digestive tract. A few other symptoms from a short transit time are electrolyte imbalances, anemia, osteoporosis, muscle cramps, etc.

A research conducted on 21 healthy people to measure their digestion time showed an average of 39 hours, which could be due to our changing lifestyle, consumption of more processed foods than raw foods, more sedentary work styles, and many more reasons.

Anyone suffering from chronic constipation or loose stools, abdominal cramping, diarrhea, and a bowel transit time of less than 10 hours or more than 30 hours should seek the advice of a physician or a medical professional. They may suggest you to undergo certain tests to assess you for any inflammatory bowel disease, food allergies or sensitivities, ulcerative colitis, endocrine disorders, etc. The doctor may keep a record of other features of feces too, like color, texture, and consistency to know what's actually happening in your GI (gastrointestinal tract).

Remember, a healthy stool is well formed and should be eliminated without any pushing or straining.

Chapter #5: Improving Your Food Transit Time

How can you improve your food transit time?

Transit time varies from individual to individual based on their diet, metabolic rate, overall health, and activity levels. If you are worried about your bowel transit time, making small adjustments in your daily schedule can help improve your rate. Starting an exercise program or shifting to a healthy, more fibrous diet are some of the habits which one should inculcate in their routine.

The following are some of the ways you can improve your bowel transit time:

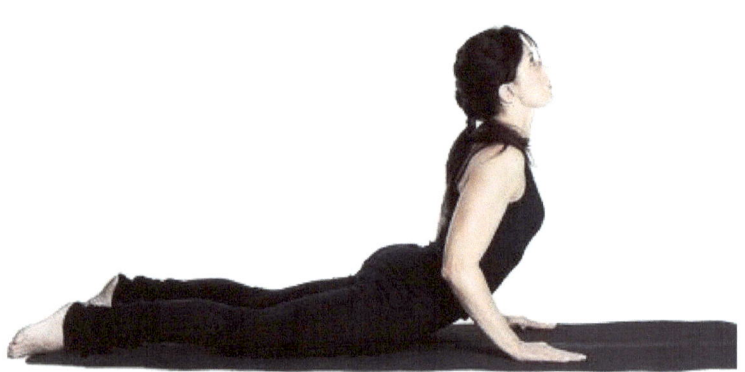

- **Exercise:** Food and digested material in our digestive tract, moves through a series of muscle contractions called peristalsis. A sedentary lifestyle slows the process of peristalsis and thus decreases transit time.

So, it is important to indulge in any light exercise of at least 30 minutes daily, like walking, doing breathing exercises, or light stretching exercises.

- **Diet:** Fiber is a very essential component of any diet. One should consume around 30 to 40 grams of fiber daily. This may include fresh fruits, leafy vegetables, whole grains, etc. Fiber stimulates the muscle contractions and pushes the food along the digestive tract. If you consume very low amounts of fiber, try to increase your fiber intake gradually. Adding too much fiber too quickly in your diet may result in uncomfortable symptoms, like abdominal cramps, gas, and bloating. Also, avoid soda drinks and drink less of coffee and tea.

- **Water intake:** Drink at least eight glasses of water daily, if you lead a normal active life. If you exercise or sweat a lot, drink more to keep yourself hydrated and your stools moist.

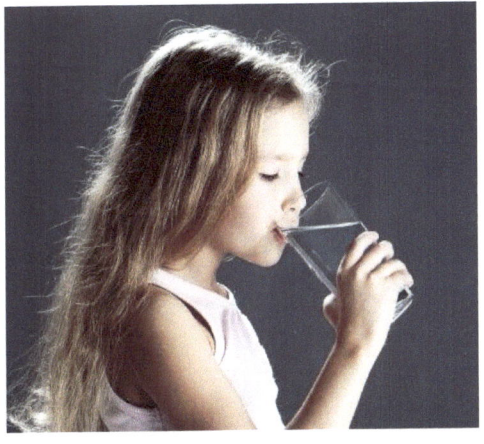

More water content in the body improves the transit time through your digestive tract. Also, if you see your urine color is dark yellow or brown, it's an indication that your body is dehydrated.

Caution: If you are already undergoing any medication for bowel disorder, it's better to consult your doctor before making any changes in your diet.

Also, there may be an initial period of a week or two when one may experience more gas and bloating, as your body is adjusting to the change in pH levels of your intestine. But, do not worry, because once the body adjusts, your stomach will be flatter and there will be no gas or bloating.

Learning Tips and Tricks for Controlled Eating

Chapter #6: Tips for Eating Mindfully

- **Choose the right place:** Eating in a place free of any distraction, such as the TV, phone, newspaper, or computer is very important. This is because, when you eat with all the distractions around, your mind focuses more on the distractions than on eating. This may make you feel full but not satisfied. Indulging in these distractions while eating, makes your brain delay or skip sending the signal of fullness, thus resulting in overeating or unsatisfied eating.

- **Choose the right posture:** It is best to eat while sitting down at a dining table or on floor, instead of sitting on a couch or bed or while standing near the refrigerator or kitchen.

- **Choose the right food:** Choose food that satisfies both the body and mind. Often, we are so obsessed with eating right that we eat things we don't even like. These things make us full, but we miss the pleasure of eating our favorite foods. Feeling guilty about eating certain foods may actually cause more overeating. If while eating anything, you feel that you are not enjoying it, it's better to choose something else. Eating foods without pleasure will leave an unsatisfying feeling after your meal.

- **Appreciate the environment:** Appreciate the ambience, the atmosphere, the company of family and friends, or simply the fact that one has given themselves the opportunity to sit down peacefully and enjoy a meal.

- **Acknowledge the food:** Smell the aroma, notice the appearance, the color, the texture of the food, and imagine its taste. Always go for the quality of the food instead of the quantity. Selecting small portions of the best quality food will add to its affordability, will add to the pleasure of eating, and will satisfy the inner self, automatically.

- **Appreciate the food:** Appreciate the food while eating. Put the cutlery down between bites and concentrate on each different sensation of the food you experience. Focus on how much you like or dislike these sensations. Look for the most appetizing food and start with it first, because if that is kept for the end, you are sure to overeat and stuff yourself with it.

- **Pause while eating:** Before starting the meal, just take a deep breath and thank God that He has given you this opportunity to enjoy your meal. This practice will help in initiating the focus to the pleasure of eating. Between bites, concentrate on chewing your food. Take smaller portions to eat and if possible put down the cutlery between bites. Pause in the middle of eating and estimate how much more is required to satisfy your hunger.

- **Push plate forward when done:** Once the practice of pushing the plate forward is inculcated, the desire to eat more will pass quickly. Just keep in mind that whenever you are hungry you'll eat again.

- **Prepare mindful food:** You should take time to prepare your own meals, preferably from fresh ingredients. The cooking process can be as relaxing and enjoyable as eating. When we know what ingredients have been used for cooking the food and how they were cleaned and utilized, we automatically feel more satisfied and enjoy our food.

Once this concept is practiced, one is sure to learn the real meaning of "Mindful Eating."

The experience of increased pleasure and satisfaction of mindful eating may motivate a person to become more mindful for other activities too. Being aware of living "in the moment" cannot only increase the enjoyment and satisfaction, but even the effectiveness in every task that is performed.

Chapter #7: Five Tricks to Keep Your Stomach Happy for Hours

Trick #1: Eat foods with a high water content

The best zero calorie food, is water! Since it is a liquid, it takes up a good quantity of your stomach, making you feel full. Most nutritionists suggest drinking water before you eat, for this reason. About 15 minutes before you eat a meal, drink 16 ounces of water, this will help you eat less, because the water makes you feel full, and thus eating less calories.

Another strategy, when you do eat choose foods with a higher water content. Fruits and vegetables are mainly comprised of water, where pastas and breads have very little water content.

You can feel more satiated by eating 100 calories of grapes (a small bowl full) than with 100 calories from raisins (a quarter cup), since grapes have 6 times more water than raisins.

Salads having cucumbers, lettuce, and tomatoes have high water content (it's full of vegetables), the same is true for broth based soups. This is why starting your meal with a salad or soup will also help you in consuming fewer calories, you will feel fuller faster.

Also, an ideal between meal snack could be whole fruit rather than dried fruit, which apart from having fewer calories, is more satiating.

Tip #2: Eat foods with high fiber content

Foods higher in glucose are going to be absorbed into the bloodstream faster, making you feel hungry much sooner.

Food that is high in fiber, is not going to convert to glucose very fast. This will help you feel full longer, fiber acts just like water, in the sense that it fills up space in your stomach without adding calories.

Apart from that, fiber has some hidden benefits that are very helpful when you are trying to consume fewer calories. Firstly, when you consume fiber and fluids together, the fiber soaks up water and gets even fluffier. It also slows down the speed at which the food leaves your stomach, giving the feeling of fullness for a longer period of time. When the food travels into the small intestine, the fiber in foods stimulate the release of a hormone that sends a signal of satiation to the brain.

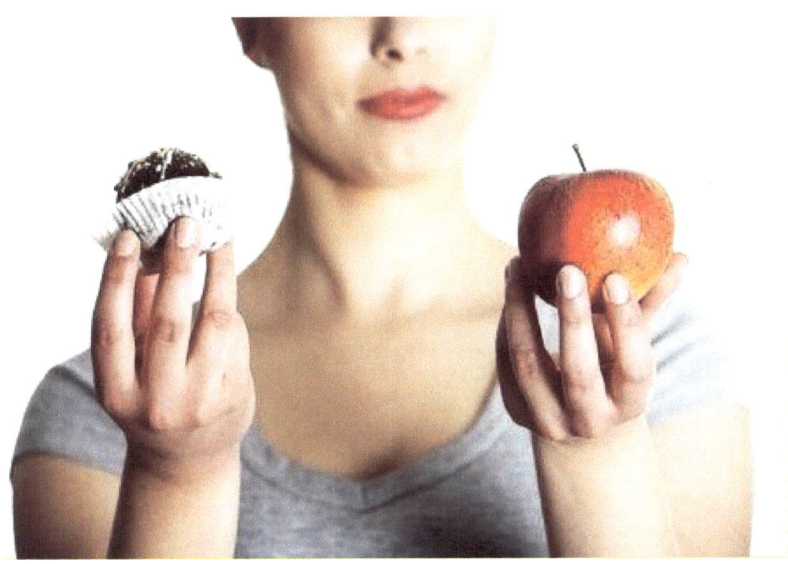

Foods rich in fiber are vegetables, whole grains, bran, fruits, etc. So, try including a high fiber cereal in your breakfast that will keep you feeling fuller longer than a low fiber cereal (usually these are high glucose). Also, a cup of black bean soup will give you more fullness than a cup of mushroom cream soup.

Tip #3: Add more proteins than starches to your diet

Another major factor that regulates the appetite is how fast the blood sugar rises and falls after a meal. Carbohydrates are broken down into glucose at a faster rate than proteins and fats. A high protein diet keeps you full for longer, as it requires many digestive steps to get converted and digested.

For example, instead of a chicken sandwich with two slices of bread and a slice of chicken, opt for an open sandwich with one slice bread and two slices of chicken. Though both of them have about the same number of calories, the higher protein portion—more chicken slices—will keep you full and satisfied for longer.

During breakfast too, opt for an extra egg and one fewer piece of toast. While snacking, instead of having handful of pretzels, it's better to have a few pretzels and some cheese.

Trick #4: Use smaller plates and bowls for eating and large glasses for drinking water

Delboeùf illusion says that if we put two circles of the same size close to each other (say our food), then surround one by a large ring (think a large plate), and the other by a smaller ring (think a small plate), it makes the circle surrounded by the large ring appear to be smaller.

Therefore, we usually end up serving ourselves more than if we served our food on a small plate.

On the contrary, use large glasses to drink water so that consumption of one glass of water gives more water content to our body and makes us feel full.

Trick #5: End with tea

A mug of hot tea after a meal helps in suppressing one's appetite. For example, green tea contains a phytonutrient that increases the level of a hormone that triggers the feeling of satiation and sends a signal of fullness to the brain.

Similarly, having mint tea after a meal can help in suppressing the unwanted craving of having more food.

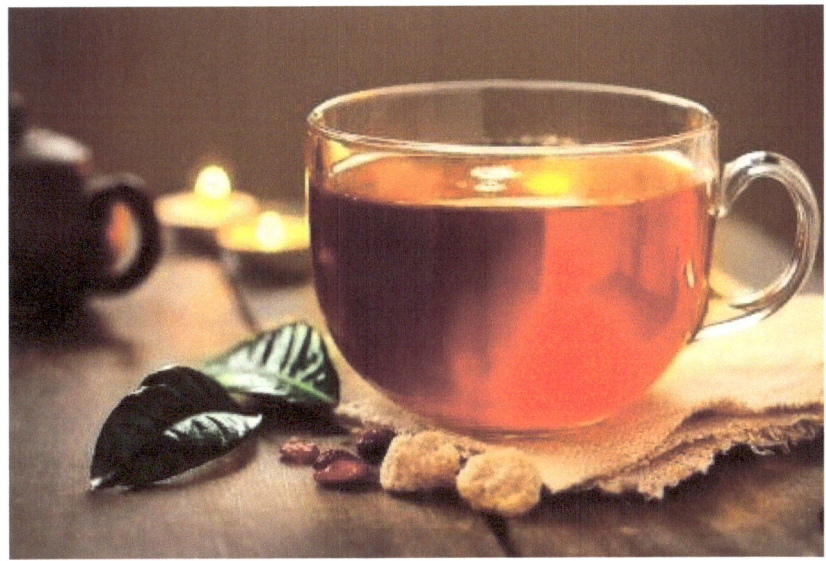

Mindful Workout

Chapter #8: Techniques/Exercises for Practicing a Mindful Workout

The basic principle of doing a mindful workout is to be "present in the moment." It's no wonder our minds wander, but the effort should be put in to bring back our mind to the task we are performing. This requires practice and is very easily achievable with dedication and patience.

Let's try the following exercises to get started:

Exercise # 1: Observation and patience

Observe:

Perform this exercise prior to having your meal.

+ Select your food and put it on the plate.

+ Take a deep breath (inhale till the belly extends and exhale through the mouth).

+ Focus your eyes and mind on the food.

+ Observe each food item and examine its contents.

+ Close your eyes.

+ Inhale the smell of the food and exhale.

Patience:

+ Sit quietly and take few deep breaths.

- Select a food or a drink: One can select anything that they like to eat/drink for that moment; be it a fruit, a raisin, a chocolate shake, bread, etc.

- Take a smaller potion, i.e. a slice of fruit, 3-4 raisins, a piece of bread, or a quarter of a drink, etc.

- Take a bite/sip: Take your first bite/sip and keep it in your mouth for a minute, just feeling it with the tongue and teeth.

- Close your eyes and observe anything that comes to mind: the taste and the sensation.

- Start chewing your food. Chew it for few minutes. Notice every movement of the jaw and throat, how the salivary glands are working, and try to hold the mind back to the task.

- Slowly observe the transition from chewing to swallowing.

- Notice the way the food/drink travels through the mouth to the throat.

- Keep track of the food/drink till there is no sensation.

- Take a deep breath and exhale.

- Repeat the process a couple of times.

How does it feel?

The purpose of this exercise is not to eat our meals in this manner all the time, but to gain an insight about our eating habits, and where we stand in our relationship with the food consumed. These exercises not only draw our awareness to mind-body connection, but also help us in knowing how we put food into our body.

Though, initially, this exercise might seem very boring and redundant, with practice and time, it is sure to make eating more enjoyable and satisfying.

To start with, it's better to perform this exercise to every first bite of each meal. This will help in setting an intention of being mindful throughout the course of the meal.

Exercise # 2: Follow the 80-20 rule:

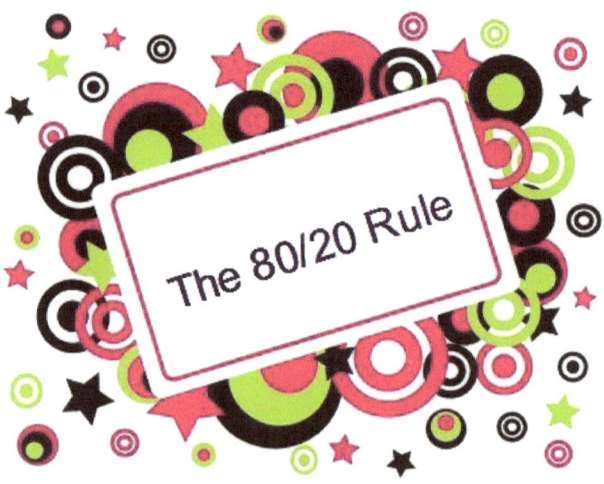

This rule instructs you to stop eating when 80 percent of our hunger is satisfied. It has been scientifically proven that it takes around 20 minutes for our stomach to send a signal to our brain that it is full. In those 20 minutes, whatever is consumed is just a part of overeating. It's no surprise that people who consume their meals quickly are habitual overeaters.

Exercise # 3: Break the meals:

This exercise/technique instructs you to break the meal into two halves. First, consume one-half and take a few minutes break, say around 5-7 minutes, and then start eating the second half. This exercise will regulate the pace of your eating and will help us in knowing the extent of our hunger. Since there is a delay in our stomach knowing that it is full and our brain knowing that the stomach is full, this pace regulating exercise will help a lot in avoiding any overeating.

Exercise # 4: Eat with the non-dominant hand:

It's always better to eat with the non-dominant hand, while learning mindful eating. Having to work harder to hold the utensils will automatically make the eating process slow and bring a whole new awareness to eating mindfully and avoiding any overeating.

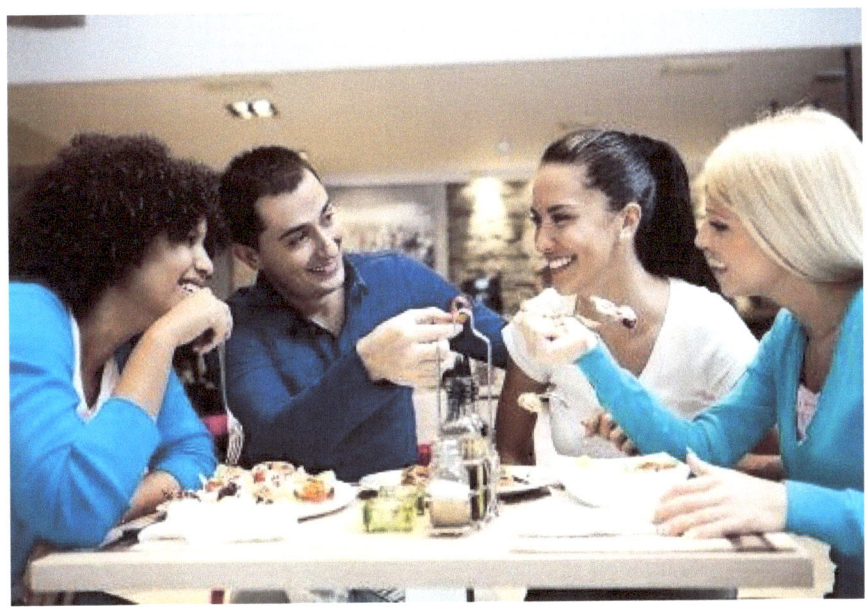

Exercise # 5: Slow eating race:

This exercise can be performed with like-minded people, in which, one can compete with others to finish the meal last; pausing in between for conversations about the food, its taste, its texture, likes, and dislikes. Though, initially, it may seem a bit weird, eventually this exercise can turn out to be really fun and informative.

Exercise # 6: Chew more:

One of the most common overlooked parts of eating is chewing. Chewing takes time, and time facilitates fullness. Mindful chewing is a very nice way to slow down the whole eating process. Though many people suggest chewing a particular food for "X" number of times, the best way for effective chewing is to observe the whole process of chewing. Notice the side of the mouth one chews on or count the number of chewing motions per bite. Feel what it is to keep food in the mouth and not chew it for a moment. Observe how it feels after we have chewed the food enough. What is the sensation and how do we know that it's time to swallow the food?

This exercise will not only help in inculcating a better chewing habit that can be easily digested by our digestive system, but it will also help in eating to an extent when our stomach is full, thus avoiding overeating.

Exercise # 7: Resting hands:

You should rest your hands between bites, i.e. lay down your silverware and rest your hands on the table after each bite. This will greatly help in slowing down your pace of eating and give time for the brain to send the signal of fullness at the right time.

To get into the habit of resting your hands, try placing to bells on either side of your plate, where your hands would naturally rest. When one rests their hands on the sides, they hear a ringing tone as the hands touch the bells.

What do you do during the pause? Just take a breath and listen to the fading sound of the bell. Wait to eat another bite until the sound has faded into silence.

Exercise # 8: Count the chips:

Look at the bag of chips, before you eat, and make a prediction on the number of chips you think will be in the bag. Then, count the chips while you are eating them. If the bag is not finished (which is shouldn't be in one sitting), write down the number on the bag with a marker and continue counting the next time. When the bag is finished, compare the actual results with the prediction you made.

Even if your prediction was way off, this exercise is surely a fun way to help slow down your pace and increase the consciousness of eating by preventing a sense of disappointment. This technique can be applied to any finger-food, snack, or sweet (which happens to be the foods we most overeat, hence the name "mindless snaking").

Exercise # 9: Reminiscence eating:

Eating often links people, places, and things of our pasts. Reminiscent eating is a great way to re-associate with the past, by observing the dish and relating it to any dish which one has tasted or smelled in the past. It thus helps in slowing down the process of eating and making the simple act of eating turn into a sentimental, meaningful and mindful experience.

Conclusion:

There is no "right" or "wrong" way of doing any mindful eating exercise. If, in spite of all the effort, you still feel that your mind is busy thinking of something else while performing these exercises, there is no need to panic.

You have still learned something useful about how mindless or unconscious eating is a part of your daily routine, and how easy it can be to gobble your food, even when you are attempting to eat mindfully.

Performing these exercises once a day will change your experience from mindless gobbling to mindful eating.

Mindfulness is just like a muscle that might be weak initially, but with regular practice, it will become strong and more readily available.

Our physical, mental, emotional, and psychological survival depends a lot on our regular intake of food, water, light, sound, and love from our environments. How well or poorly we relate to these things will determine how happy or unhappy we are in our lives.

Mindful eating helps us to let go of our unhealthy relationship with food and eating and replaces it with healthy alternatives. With mindful attention to our eating habits, one can break the guilt and dissatisfaction of food and begin to cultivate the pleasure and satisfaction of eating.

Remember, it's always better to practice "Mindful eating than Mind-full eating."

References

http://www.quickanddirtytips.com/health-fitness/healthy-eating/3-tips-on-how-to-eat-less-without-feeling-hungry

http://zenhabits.net/mindful-eating/

http://eatingmindfully.com/mindful-eating/

Author Bio

Muhammad Usman is a distinguished medical graduate of Allama Iqbal medical college (AIMC). He is a professional writer who has been in the field for more than 4 years. During this time he has produced 10,000+ articles, blogs, and eBooks on various niches related to diseases, health, fitness, nutrition, and well-being. He is a regular contributor to several journals related to medicine and surgery. He is the editor of several journals and newspapers.

Check out some of the other JD-Biz Publishing books
Gardening Series on Amazon

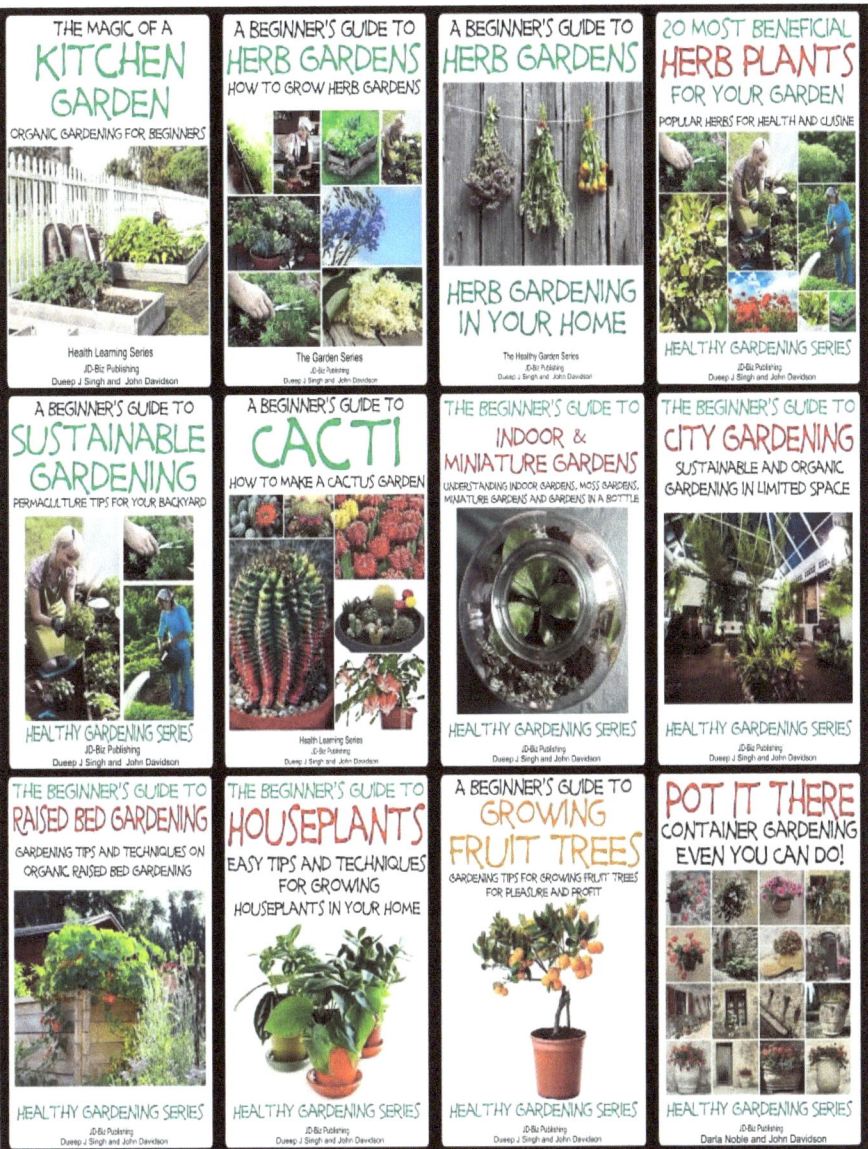

Health Learning Series

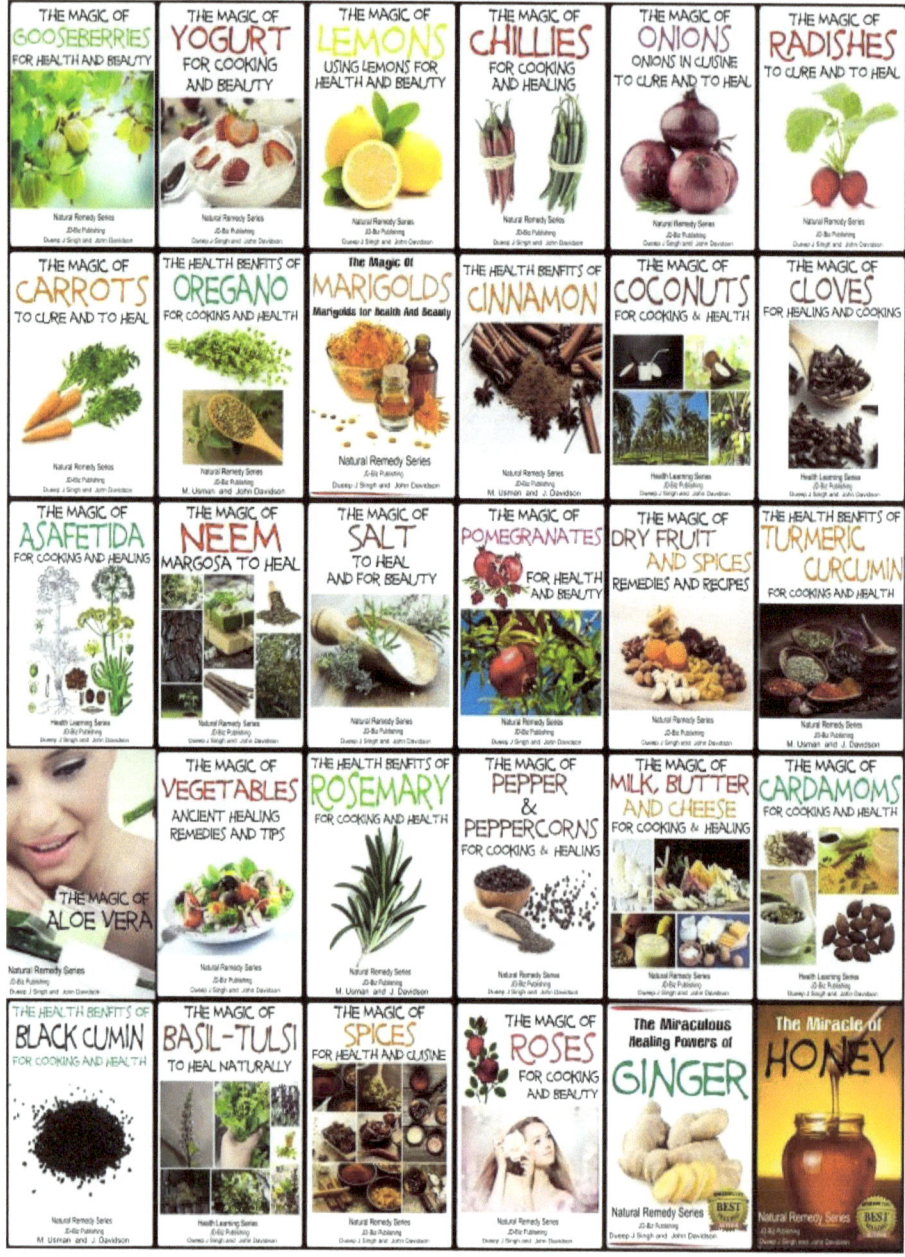

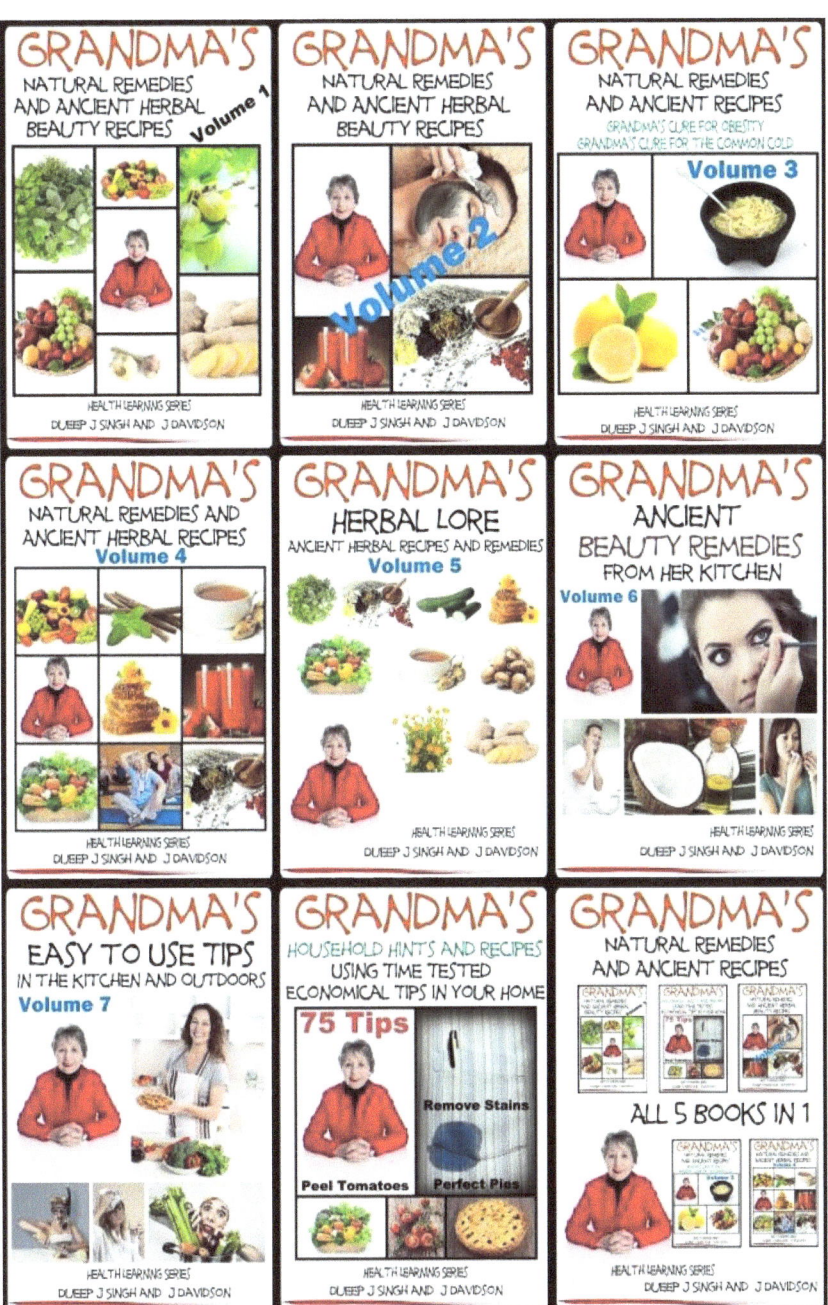

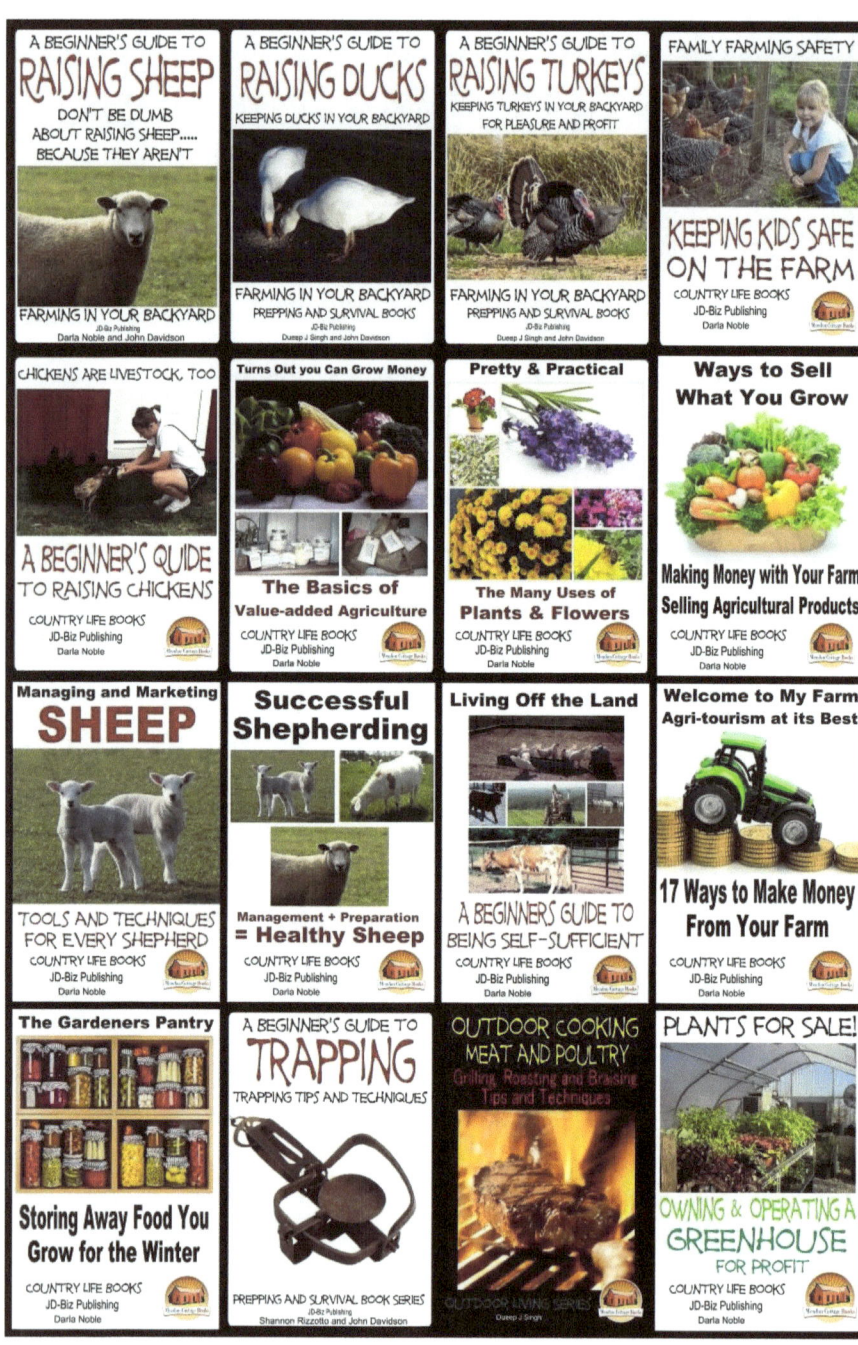

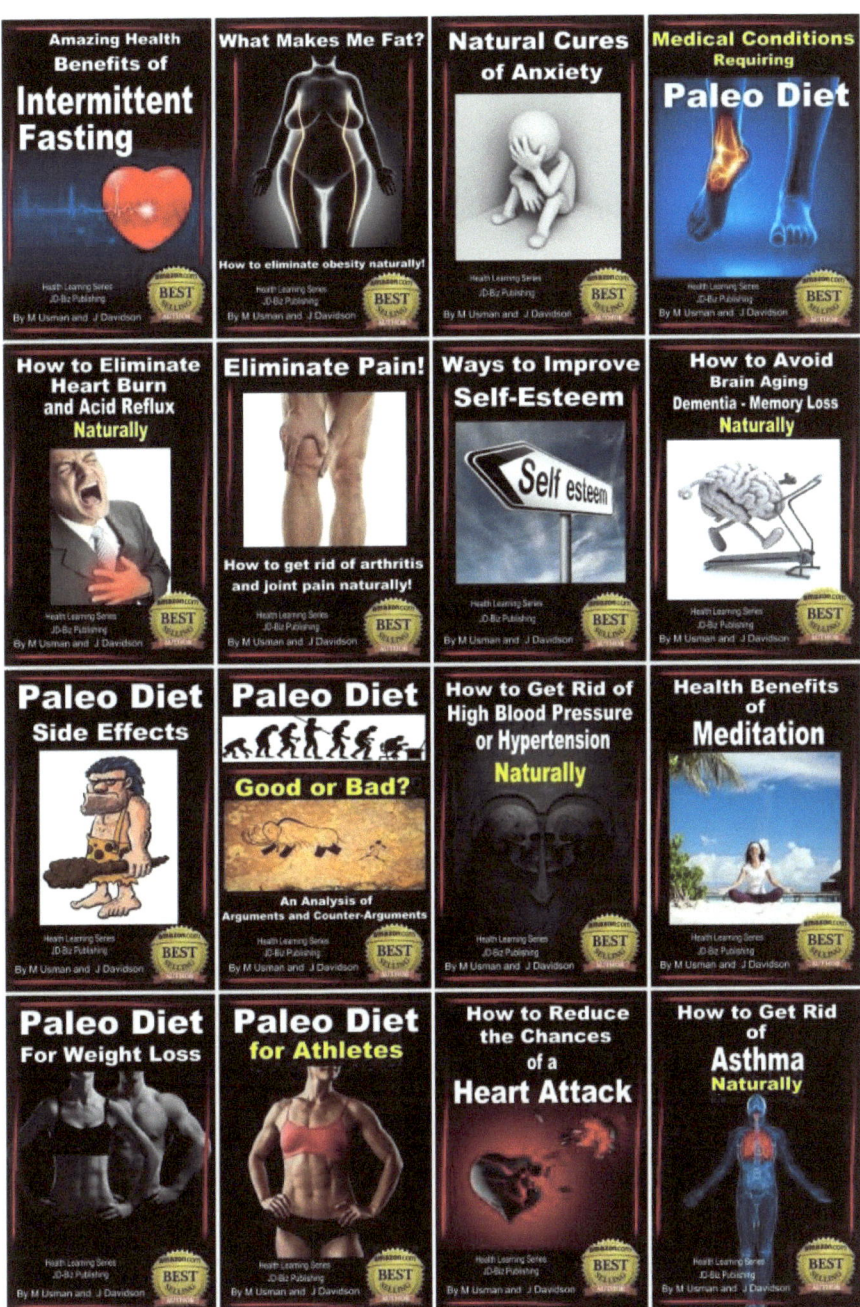

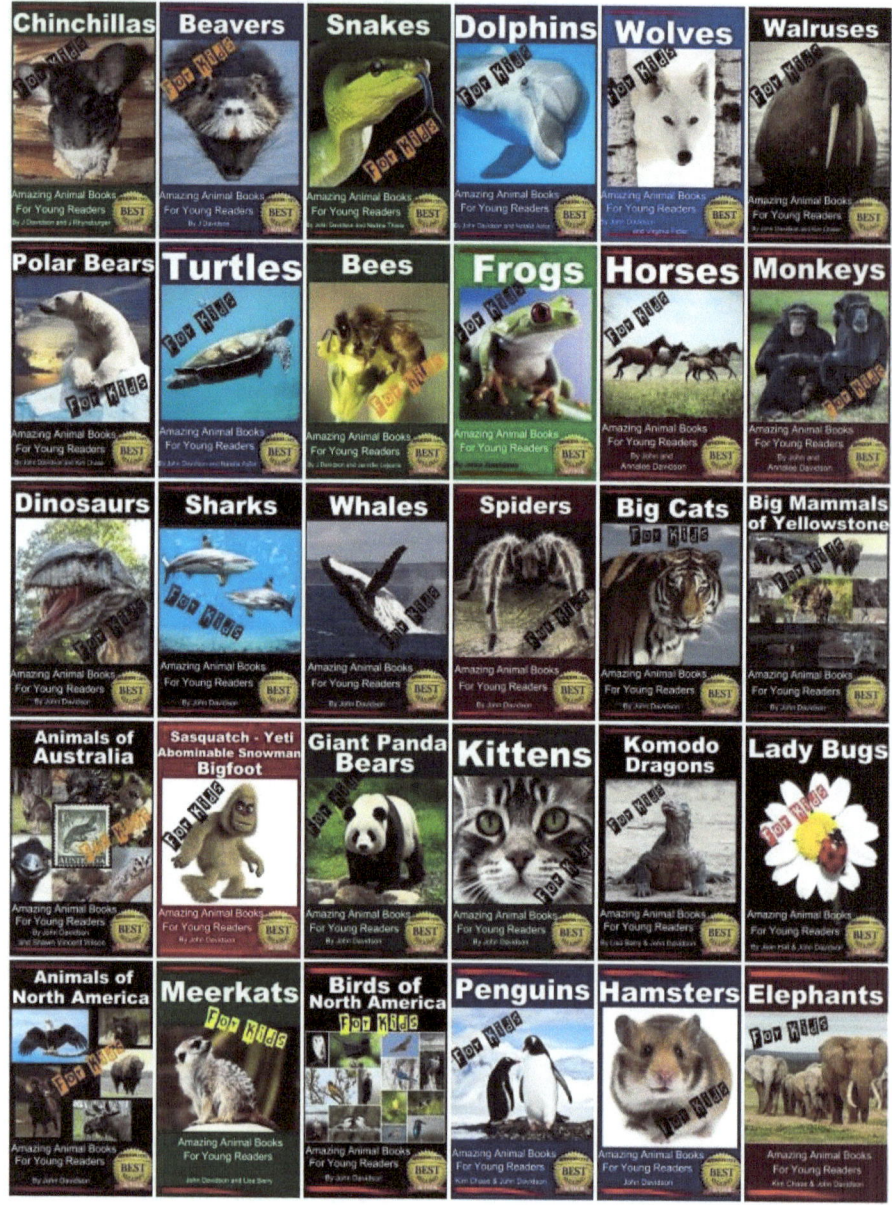

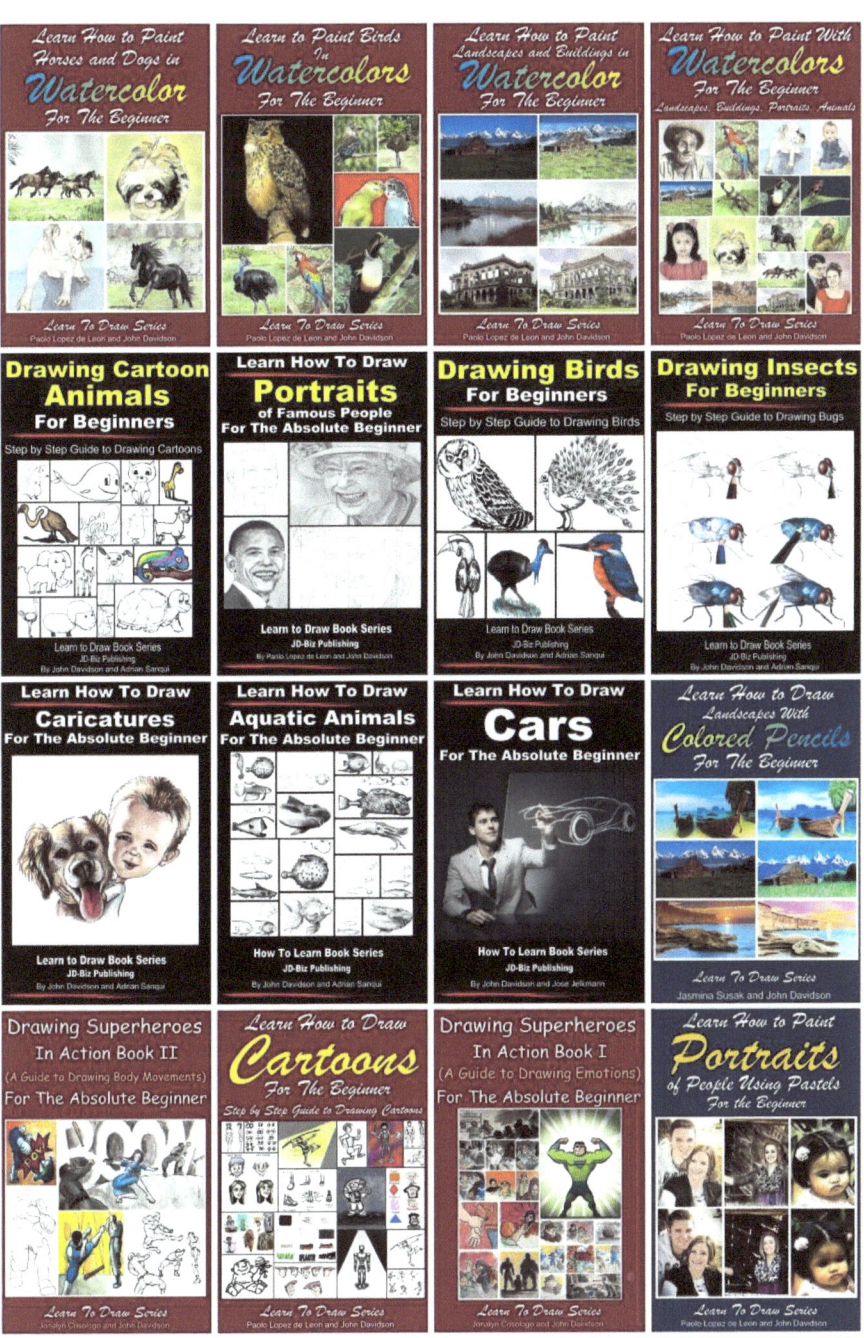

How to Build and Plan Books

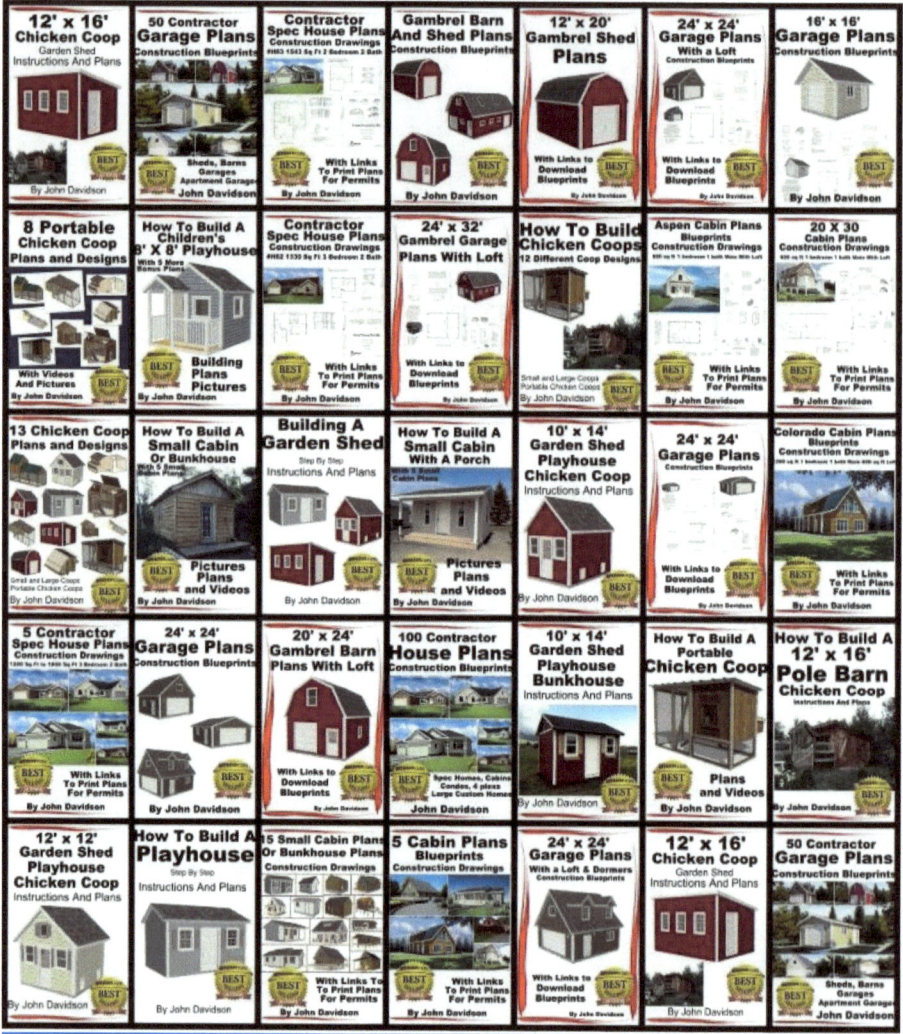

Entreprenuer Book Series

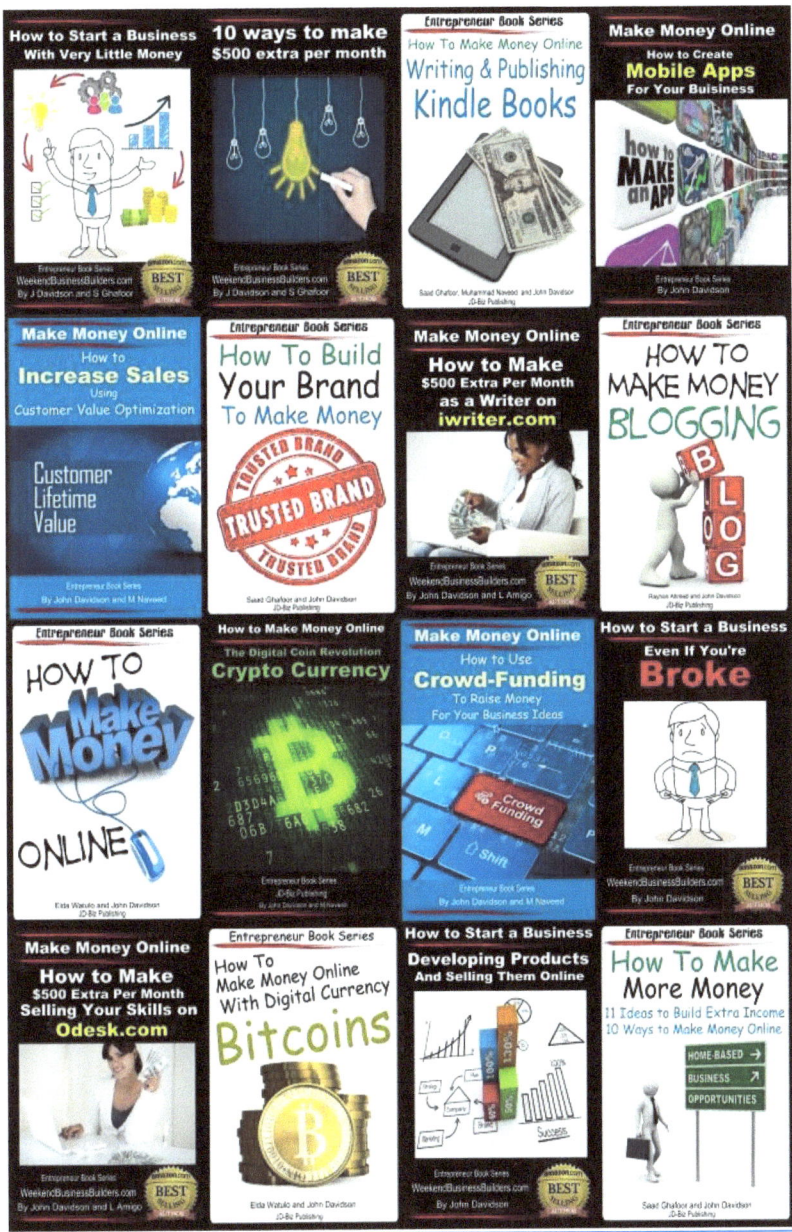

Our books are available at

1. Amazon.com

2. Barnes and Noble

3. Itunes

4. Kobo

5. Smashwords

6. Google Play Books

Download Free Books!
http://MendonCottageBooks.com

Publisher

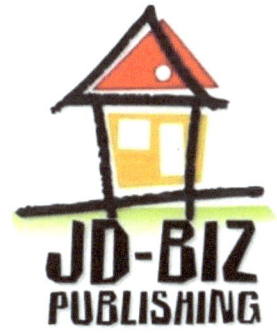

JD-Biz Corp

P O Box 374

Mendon, Utah 84325

http://www.jd-biz.com/

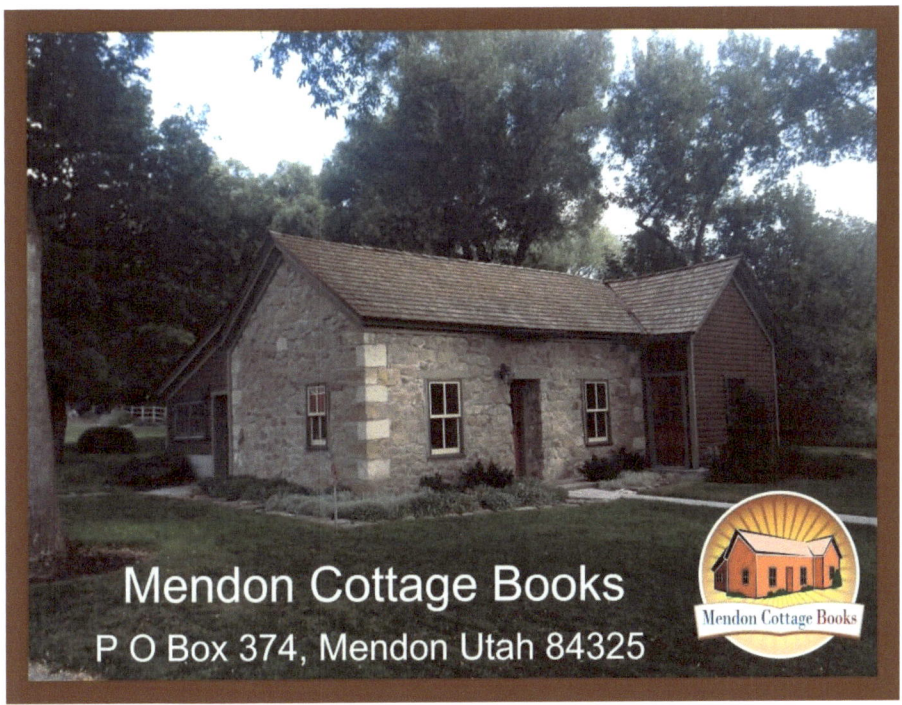

www.ingramcontent.com/pod-product-compliance
Lightning Source LLC
Chambersburg PA
CBHW050845290526
45792CB00002B/532